Conquer Your A-fib
How to Beat Atrial Fibrillation

by Lisa M. White

Table of Contents

My A-Fib Story

Like most people, I can vividly recall my first a-fib episode. It was an ordinary June day in 2001 and I was working in my home office. The mail arrived, the dog barked and startled me. Bending down to pick up the post, I suddenly felt my heart take off at a hundred miles per hour, beating wildly and dramatically in the craziest of rhythms. I felt dizzy and light headed and everything became very surreal. Thoughts rushed through my mind – am I having a heart attack? A stroke? Is this the "big one"?

A few minutes earlier I had been a relatively healthy 31-year-old female with no known heart issues and now I felt sure I was about to imminently expire! Instead of going straight to the accident and emergency department, I sought an emergency appointment with my GP. An hour later I was sat in her office with my heart still beating madly out of control, my adrenaline rising and having an intense desire to rush to the toilet every few minutes.

My doctor confirmed that my heart was indeed racing at about 150 BPM and an ECG revealed that whatever was going on was supra-ventricular. "What does that mean?" I asked nervously. "It means that it isn't going to kill you" she replied. Well that was reassuring I suppose!

I was sent to the local hospital in a taxi rather than an ambulance since it was confirmed that my demise had been postponed, with a differential diagnosis of supra-ventricular tachycardia/atrial fibrillation/atrial flutter. About half way to the hospital I felt my heart
rhythm change, no longer did it feel that a mule was trying to kick its way out of my chest although I did still feel anxious and light-headed. On arrival in the emergency department, I was hooked up to an ECG which revealed my heart was now

beating normally, although the rate was still a little high at 110-120 bpm. This was no doubt due to the adrenaline which was now circulating through my veins due to the events of the morning.

The National Health Service here in England is nothing if not thorough at times, even if they had lost the original print out from my ECG at the doctor's office. Three days in the hospital and a barrage of tests revealed a whole list of conditions that I did not have, and nothing conclusive to explain what I did have. An echo-cardiogram found that there was nothing structurally wrong with my heart, and a consultant cardiologist even complimented me on my good heart function. I had not had a heart attack, my bloods were perfect, my ECG was normal and my thyroid was fine. I was a medical mystery!

Three days later, a doctor came and sat beside my bed. "We think we know what you have" she said. "Don't worry, it is not life threatening and we can control it". She went on to explain how they thought I had a condition called paroxysmal atrial fibrillation. Whilst it is often connected to heart problems, in some people without underlying cardiac disease it "just happened". Unfortunately, I was one of those people. I had lone a-fib and no-one had any answers. What I did learn was that a-fib was uncommon in younger people and even less common in women. "Why me?" was my immediate question. "We just don't know" said the doctors. I was told to go away, life my life and stop worrying. "A-fib won't kill you", said the doctors. "In fact you have much the same life expectancy as the general population".

Not worrying is not something I am particularly good at, and when I got home I consulted Dr Google. That was a mistake. Up until that time, no-one had mentioned that I could be at risk of stroke or heart failure. In fact, no-one had mentioned that a-fib was particularly serious at all. In 2001, the main hope for a cure lay with the Maze procedure which involved open heart surgery or an experimental ablation technique which was very much in its infancy. Everything I read on a-fib was scary, and predicted that within 15 years my atrial fibrillation would have progressed from paroxysmal to permanent. Everything seemed to be doom and gloom

Well nearly 15 years on and I'm here to tell you that none of those predictions have come true. A-fib can be conquered and overcome. Over the past 14 years, I have had many episodes of a-fib, some lasting just a few seconds and some lasting over 9 hours. It didn't progress to permanent a-fib or even get significantly worse. Eventually, I cracked what was causing it in my particular case and that solved it for me. I take no drugs, have had no surgery and a-fib no longer has that horrible control over my life it once did have. I have not seen a doctor about a-fib for over 5 years and I remain in perfect sinus rhythm.

If you are battling a-fib take heart (excuse the bad pun!). In the past one and a half decades, massive strides have been made in curing this life-destroying affliction. Although a-fib may not be life threatening it can put a huge burden on your quality of life and mental health. Nearly a third of people with a-fib suffer from depression and anxiety about their condition.

The strategies and information in this book will help you, and you could find information that your doctors or the drug companies may not tell you. It draws from both clinical studies and the experiences of people who are actually living with a-fib.   The disorder is a challenge for doctors to treat effectively, and it also requires patients to be proactive and willing to do some detective work to determine any potential triggers or leads. The idea is to figure out what works for you. For some people this may be natural remedies. For some lifestyle changes may be all that is needed. Others may choose to have an ablation.   Either way the goal is to restore normal sinus rhythm and reclaim your life. Don't let a-fib destroy your life. It doesn't have to.

Wishing you the very best health.

What is Atrial Fibrillation?

Atrial fibrillation is the most common arrhythmia, caused by disordered electrical signals in the heart. The adult heart normally beats at around 60-100 bpm in a smooth, organised manner known as sinus rhythm. In a-fib this rhythm is disrupted by errant electrical impulses, which cause the heart to beat rapidly and irregularly at up to 180 beats per minute.

If you feel your pulse when you are in a-fib you will find there is no regular pattern to it. It may feel fluttery or skip beats, it may pound rapidly one moment and then pause. Doctors call this an "irregularly irregular" rhythm. As well as an erratic pulse, you may experience other symptoms such as fatigue, shortness of breath, dizziness or chest pain. Some people have no symptoms at all and a-fib is only found on a routine medical check-up.

Let's take a quick look at how the heart normally works and then look at what happens when the heart is in a-fib. The heart has four chambers – the left and right atria at the top of the heart and the left and right ventricles at the bottom of the heart. When the heart beats, an electrical impulse travels from the top to the bottom of the heart. This signal causes the heart to contract and to pump blood around the body.

A heartbeat starts in the sinoatrial node, the SA node in the right atrium. It then travels through the atria and to the AV node (atrioventricular node) between the top and the bottom of the heart. There is a slight slowing of the signal to allow the ventricles to fill with blood before it travels to the ventricles. The ventricles then contract and the blood in them is pumped through the body. Once the ventricles are empty, the next heart beat can be initiated.

In atrial fibrillation, the heartbeat is not initiated in the SA node but in another part of the atria, often around the pulmonary veins. Instead of initiating a nice steady heartbeat, the electrical signal goes haywire and floods the atria with impulses. If you have ever seen an electrical short circuit which causes a shower of sparks, this is similar to what is happening in the atria. The resulting electrical impulses cause the atria to fibrillate at up to 600 bpm. Luckily, all of those signals are not passed down to the ventricles, as the AV node cannot keep pace. If it could the heart would beat at 300-600 beats per minute! Instead only some of the signals are passed down to the ventricles which is what causes the rapid and irregular beating of the heart in a-fib. The heart may beat at up to 180 beats per minute, and the pulse feels "irregularly irregular" as there is no pattern to the heartbeat due to the electrical storm.

As the heart cannot pump all the blood out fast enough, some of it backs up in the atria where eventually it may begin to coagulate and cause a clot. (See the chapter Atrial Fibrillation and Stroke).   This is why doctors often recommend blood thinning medication for people with a-fib as it can significant reduce the chances that a clot will form.   However, not everyone with atrial fibrillation is at high risk of stroke. Several studies have found that people with lone a-fib and no other risk factors have no significantly greater chance of a stroke than the general population. Nevertheless, anyone with atrial fibrillation should speak to their doctors about their individual risk factors and a decision made on whether anti-coagulation is necessary.

Atrial fibrillation can be a frightening disorder to live with, it is not usually considered life threatening. The pumping capacity of the heart is reduced by 10-30% and for most people this will lead to relatively minor symptoms such as fatigue and exercise intolerance.
Many people live for years in permanent a-fib and live happy and productive lives. Nevertheless, with the new advances in medical and natural treatment for a-fib, what was once seen as a chronic disorder can now be effectively cured for many patients.

What Causes A-Fib?

A-fib can be caused by many things, from structural disorders of the heart to overindulgence in alcohol (the so-called holiday heart syndrome).   Some of the most common causes of a-fib include :

Problems with the structure of the heart, particularly the valves.
Hypertension – high blood pressure.
Coronary artery disease
Previous heart attack
Congenital heart defects
Thyroid imbalance
Obesity
Lung disorders
Stimulants – alcohol, caffeine, nicotine, illegal drugs, overeating
Heart surgery
Mineral deficiencies – especially magnesium and potassium
Sleep apnoea
Physical and mental stress
Viruses
Diabetes
Prescription drug side effects.

For some people a-fib has no apparent cause. This is known as lone a-fib – atrial fibrillation which occurs in a structurally normal heart with none of the traditional risk factors. Lone A-fib is associated with a very low risk of complication including stroke. Between 10 and 20% of people who have a-fib have lone a-fib. It is quite common in athletes and other people in peak physical fitness, although no-one knows why. It has been postulated that lone a-fib may be caused by mineral deficiency caused by the body using additional resources during endurance activity. It has also been attributed to dietary factors such as wheat or gluten intolerance or a sensitivity to tyramine – a chemical which is found in cheese and red wine. We will look more at a-fib and how it is affected by diet later.

Classification of Atrial Fibrillation

Atrial fibrillation can be classified into three categories – paroxysmal, persistent and permanent.

Paroxysmal AF
Paroxysmal A-fib is episodic and episodes last anything from a few seconds to a week or more and terminate on their own. Usually paroxysmal AF self terminates within 48 hours. Lone a-fib generally falls into this category, as lone a-fib is less likely to progress to permanent. Most a-fib starts out as paroxysmal and for some people it will not progress any further, although episodes may get longer as time goes on.

Persistent AF
Persistent a-fib continues for more than 7 days consistently, with no normal sinus rhythm in between. Persistent a-fib will often not terminate on its own, so doctors may attempt to restore sinus rhythm by means of drugs or an electrical cardioversion – an electric shock designed to terminate the rhythm and restore a normal heartbeat.

Permanent AF
In permanent a-fib, the irregular rhythm is present all the time and no attempt is made to bring the patient into normal rhythm. Long-standing permanent a-fib is when this rhythm has persisted for over one year.

Atrial fibrillation was once considered to be a progressive disease, which started off as paroxysmal and then progressed to be a full time rhythm. Fifteen years was thought to be the magical number in which time most cases progressed to permanent. However, many patients (myself included) proved that this is not the case. It is often stated that "a-fib begets a-fib" meaning that the longer one stays in a-fib the more likely that electrical remodelling of the heart will occur making a-fib easier to induce. However, an interesting study using goat hearts (M Wijffels et al) found that many of the electrical changes in the heart caused by inducing AF had reversed after one week in sinus rhythm.

Nevertheless, as atrial fibrillation is an uncomfortable rhythm to be in, it makes sense to terminate episodes as quickly as possible.

How Is Atrial Fibrillation Diagnosed?

A doctor may suspect a-fib from feeling your pulse or listening to your heart with a stethoscope. In a-fib the beat is always "irregularly irregular" although if your a-fib comes and goes this your heart may be beating regularly at the time of the examination.

An ECG taken during an a-fib episode is the most accurate way of diagnosing this arrhythmia. A-fib is very easy to spot on an ECG characterised by an absence of P waves and the irregular ventricular rhythm.

Catching a-fib on an ECG may prove tricky if your episodes are quite far apart and terminate quickly. Many patients have told of episodes which terminate on the steps of the hospital emergency department and the frustrations of trying to get them documented!

To capture an event, you may be asked to wear a Holter monitor or event monitor. A Holter monitor records the entire electrical activity of the heart for a set period – usually 24 to 48 hours. Electrodes are placed on your chest and you will be able to go about your daily business as normal. If your a-fib episodes are further apart, an event recorder may be used. Unlike a Holter monitor this does not record your heartbeat for the entirety, but if you feel an episode starting you press a button on the unit to record it.

What Other Tests May Be Ordered.

As a-fib may be associated with structural heart disease, an echocardiogram may be ordered. This is a painless test which uses sound waves to look at the structure and function of your heart.   An echo gives a clear picture of the valves and structure of the heart, check for enlargement (a common trigger for a-fib) and assess how well it is working.   Rarely a TEE (trans-oesophageal echo-cardiogram) may be used. This uses a small tube which is passed down your throat into the oesophagus. This allows the technician to check for blood clots in the atria and is sometimes used before a cardioversion is attempted.

Chest X-rays will usually be taken to check for any enlargement of the heart or problems in the lungs. Blood may be also taken to evaluate thyroid function and electrolyte imbalances.

What Are the Complication of A-fib?

If left untreated, a-fib can increase the risk of stroke and heart failure.   The good news is that those risk factors can be effectively managed by appropriate treatment. Those with a-fib and no structural heart problems or risk factors (lone a-fib) have a very low risk of complications, in several studies this was found to be not significantly higher than that of an age matched population.   A-fib does statistically increase the possibility of stroke or heart failure, but statistics take into account an aged population with multiple risk factors.   A-fib is by no means a death sentence, and it is very possible to live a long and normal life even in permanent a-fib. However, that certainly does not mean that any risk factors should not be addressed or that a-fib should go untreated.

Every a-fib patient should know their CHADS2 score or CHAD2SVASC score. This is a formula used by the medical profession to calculate the average risk of stroke depending on the recognised risk factors such as hypertension, diabetes, age, sex and existing heart disease. Your doctor should assess your risk and discuss the need for anti-coagulation. You may require no anti-coagulation at all, you may need to take a daily aspirin (no longer recommended in some areas) or full time anti-coagulation may be recommended. At one time, the blood thinner of choice was Warfarin but now newer drugs are on the market which do not need the regular blood tests or intensive monitoring that Warfarin requires.

When heart rates are rapid and the a-fib continues for extended periods of time, heart failure may occur, usually in patients who already have existing cardiac problems. If the heart cannot pump out enough blood because it is beating too rapidly for the ventricles to fully fill, symptoms such as fatigue and shortness of breath can occur. Blood can start to back up in the pulmonary veins which in turn leads to a fluid build-up in the lungs. Eventually fluid may also start to build up in other parts of the body such as the feet and ankles or the abdomen.

Effective treatment of a-fib can greatly reduce the chance of any complications from the disorder. Whilst you are working on eliminating your atrial fibrillation completely, ensure that in the meantime it is effectively treated.

Neurogenic A-Fib - Vagal and Adrenergic

Neurogenic A-fib describes a type of a-fib which is triggered by an imbalance of the nervous system. The autonomic nervous system or ANS is split into two branches, the sympathetic nervous system and the parasympathetic nervous system.   One of the easiest analogies to use to describe this nervous system is that the sympathetic nervous system is the accelerator of the body, whereas the parasympathetic nervous system is the brake.

Both imbalances of the sympathetic and imbalances of the parasympathetic nervous system can trigger A-Fib. Adrenergic a-fib is caused by sympathetic overdrive whereas vagal a-fib is caused by a dominant parasympathetic nervous system. Increases in vagal tone – whether sympathetic or parasympathetic shorten atrial refractory periods making the atrial tissue more excitable and likely to incite a-fib.

Adrenergic A-fib
Adrenergic a-fib is caused by stress, exercise, stimulants, emotion, exertion and anything which causes the body to increase adrenaline levels. It occurs mainly in the mornings when sympathetic tone is at its highest and almost exclusively in the day time. Beta blockers are very helpful in managing this type of A-fib.

Vagal A-fib
Vagal a-fib in contrast mainly occurs in the evenings and at night, after meals and when relaxing. It generally starts in middle age, and is more common in men that women in a ratio of 4 to 1. Bending, coughing, stretching, straining on the toilet, eating a heavy meal or even lying on your side in bed can trigger it. Vagal a-fib generally lasts a few hours and terminates on its own, often in the very early morning when sympathetic tone once again becomes dominant. The good news is that this type of a-fib almost never occurs in a

structurally diseased heart and very rarely progresses to permanent. Beta blockers are not recommended for vagal a-fibbers because they can increase parasympathetic tone and make the problem worse. Gastric problems are very common in vagal a-fibbers, and it is suggested that in the increased pressure on the vagal nerve from gas, a full stomach or GERD is the culprit in triggering attacks.

A-fib and Stroke

Stroke is the most feared and devastating complication of a-fib. A stroke can occur in a-fib if blood pools in the atria and forms a clot. Because the heart is not pumping effectively, some blood may stagnate in the atria which begins to coagulate. If this clot breaks away it can travel to the brain where is can cause an embolic stroke. It is estimated that about 15% of all strokes are caused by a-fib. Lone atrial fibrillation carries a low risk of stroke and several studies have concluded that the risk of stroke in lone a-fib and aged under 60 years is not higher than the general population.

A person's chance of stroke depends on the amount of risk factors they have. To calculate potential stroke risk doctors used the CHADS2 score or more recently the CHA2DS2 VASc score.

CHADS2

Condition	Points
Congestive Heart Failure	1
Hypertension	1
Age over 75	1
Diabetes	1
Prior Stroke or TIA	2

Under the CHADS2 system a patient can score between 0 and 6 points depending on co-existing conditions. A person with no risk factors (a score of 0) has an annual stroke risk of 1.9% whereas someone with the highest score of 6 would have an annual stroke risk in the region of 18% without anti-coagulation.

The recommendations for anti-coagulation based on the Chads2 score are:
Score 0 – no anti-coagulation or Aspirin
Score 1- Aspirin or Warfarin
Score 2 or higher – Warfarin

The newer CHA2DS2-Vasc model takes into account sex and vascular disease.

Condition	Points
Congestive Heart Failure	1
Hypertension	1
Age over 75	2
Age 65-74	1
Stroke/TIA/TE	2
Vascular Disease	1
Diabetes	1
Female	1

In the UK, the NICE guidelines recommend that no anti-coagulation is necessary for men with a score of 0 and women with a score of 1. The risk of stroke is very low and the side effects of anti-coagulation outweigh the benefits.

Men with a score of 1 may be offered anti-coagulation after a discussion of the potential risks vs benefits.

Anti-coagulation should be offered to patients with a CHA2DS2-Vasc score of 2 or more.

Anticoagulation Agents

The choice of anti-coagulant is largely a matter of individual discussion between doctor and patient. Anti-coagulation is not without risks, primarily the risk of bleeding, which may be severe. Previously low risk patients were treated with aspirin (up to 49% reduction in stroke) and higher risk patients with Warfarin, often considered the gold standard of anti-coagulation therapy. Warfarin reduces the incidence of stroke by around two thirds. Unfortunately, Warfarin can be a challenging drug for patients and doctors alike. It requires regular blood tests, close monitoring, interacts with many commonly prescribed drugs and increases the possibility of haemorrhagic stroke

Several new anticoagulant drugs have now been approved for use in A-fib which do not require the intensive monitoring of Warfarin. These include Rivaroxaban, Dabigatran and Apixaban.

Other Means of Stroke Prevention

Left Atrial Appendage Occlusion.

A high percentage of the blood clots which form in a-fib occur in the LAA, a small sac located in the left atrium. In one study, 90% of the clots which formed in non valvular a-fib occurred in the left atrial appendage whilst 50% of clots in valvular a-fib did so. It is not clear what function the LAA performs yet it is clear that in a-fib, it poses a potentially potent ability to cause embolism.

The left atrial appendage can be closed off by surgery or even amputated completely. This is a relatively new technique as is currently aimed mainly at those who cannot tolerate oral anticoagulants. The Watchman LAA closure device has been approved for use in Europe and is implanted via catheter into the heart to close off the left atrial appendage. In the Protect AF study, the Watchman device was found to have a relative risk reduction of all stroke of 32% when compared to Warfarin and a relative risk reduction of 63% for disabling stroke.

Ablation and Stroke Prevention

An interesting study carried out in 2013 found that patients who had undergone an ablation procedure for AF had similar stroke rates to people who did not have AF. Unfortunately, there does not seem to be any data on how effective the ablation procedures were in curing AF, but what was clear from the study was that patients treated with ablation were at no more risk of a stroke than those who didn't have AF. Those patients with AF who did not undergo the procedure had higher stroke rates than those who did.

How the Medical Community Addresses A-fib

A patient presenting in a-fib can be quite a diagnostic challenge for a physician. The usual approach is to look for an obvious cause, underlying heart disease, high blood pressure, thyroid disorders etc. Unfortunately, for many patients that's where the detective work stops. They are sent on their way with a prescription for anti-arrhythmic or rate control drugs and perhaps started on an anti-coagulant. If the a-fib proves really stubborn they may even be referred for an ablation procedure.

Traditional Medical Approaches

Anti-Arrhythmic Drugs
anti-arrhythmic drugs stabilize the heart tissue making abnormal heart rhythms less likely to occur. Some anti-arrhythmic drugs also block impulses through the AV node slowing the heartbeat.

Paradoxically some anti-arrhythmic drugs can also be pro-arrhythmic, and some may even predispose patients to more serious arrhythmias. Patients with paroxysmal a-fib may be suitable for a "pill in the pocket" approach which, instead of taking medication every day, they can take a single tablet when they feel an a-fib episode starting.

Common Rhythm Control Drugs

Flecainide – this is a potent anti-arrhythmic which works by blocking sodium channels in the heart. It is often used as the "pill in the pocket" approach. Flecainide should not be used in anyone who has had a previous heart attack and is recommended only for patients without structural heart disease.

Solatol – Solatol is a beta blocker which works by blocking some of the beta adrenergic receptors in the heart. This makes the heart less susceptible to the effects of adrenaline and other chemicals which could excite the heart. Beta blockers can worsen vagal a-fib whereas they are the treatment of choice for adrenergic a-fib

Propafenone
Propafenone slows the passage of sodium into the heart reducing the excitability of tissue. It also has beta blocking properties It is used mainly in paroxysmal atrial fibrillation as its effectiveness in chronic a-fib has not been established.

Amiodarone
Amiodarone is a very potent anti-arrhythmic mainly used only for life threatening ventricular arrhythmia although used occasionally for the treatment of atrial fibrillation in patients for whom other drugs have not worked. Amiodarone needs to be initiated in a hospital setting and needs to very carefully monitored as it has marked potential for pulmonary toxicity.

Dofetilide
Dofetilide is another drug which needs to be initiate in a hospital setting due to its potential for causing potentially deadly arrhythmia. It is recommended that patients are monitored as an inpatient for at least 3 days when initiating or changing dose.

Dronedarone
Dronedarone is used to prevent a-fib episodes in people with paroxysmal a-fib. It is prescribed only to people who are usually in sinus rhythm and is not recommended for permanent a-fib as it can cause problems. Dronedarone has also been reported to cause liver problems including liver failure.

Rate Control Drugs

Another strategy to control a-fib is to control the ventricular rate during an episode, bringing it down to as normal as possible. Any form of sustained tachycardia including a-fib when persisting over a long period of time can eventually weaken the heart muscle, although is most cases this is reversible when the heart rate is brought down to normal. The goal in rate control therapy therefore is not to control the arrhythmia itself but to slow the rates during an episode which lessens symptoms and increases exercise tolerance. If you have a-fib with a rapid ventricular response, then this may be the strategy your health care provider may suggest. Rate control drugs include beta blockers, calcium channel blockers and cardiac glycosides.

Ablation Procedures

In 1987 James Cox invented a surgical procedure called the Maze or Cox-Maze procedure which proved effective in stopping the errant signals which trigger a-fib. It involved cutting or suturing a pattern of lines described as a "maze" in the atria. Unfortunately, whilst proving very successful, this technique involved open heart surgery, so was only used only patients who were already undergoing procedures which required the chest wall to be open.

Doctors then started looking for an alternatively minimally invasive procedure which could mimic the efficacy of the Cox-Maze procedure. A breakthrough came in France when Michel Haïssaguerre discovered that around 90% of all a-fib was triggered in an area in or around the pulmonary veins. By isolating the pulmonary veins using radio frequency energy via a catheter they found that errant impulses could be stopped from spreading to the atria thus preventing a-fib. In some of the earliest trials they found that they could stop a-fib in 62% of patients and that they no longer required blood thinners.

Since then, catheter ablation techniques have evolved and modern methods include cryoablation (using intense cold), microwave, laser and minimally invasive surgical techniques.

Success Rates for Ablation

Ablation eliminates paroxysmal atrial fibrillation in approximately 85% of cases, although more than one procedure may be required. At five years, the number of patients still in sinus rhythm is around 52%. The success rates for permanent a-fib are slightly lower at around 50%. This data is quite old now and with the efficacy of new procedures and experienced centres, the statistics are likely to improve.

Risks of Ablation

Although ablation is minimally invasive and even considered routine in many centres, with any medical procedure there are risks. Around 1-5% of procedures involve some sort of complication which may range from relatively minor such as bruising and chest pain, through to extremely serious such as stroke, atrio-oesphageal fistula and even death. The risk of complication should be discussed extensively with your chosen practitioner, and ask for their actual data on procedural complications. If they are unwilling to provide this, choose another practitioner who is. According to generalised data, death occurs in approximately 1 in 1000 procedures. The risk of having a stroke during the procedure is between 1 in 50 and 1 in 200 but this depends on additional risk factors such as age, existing heart disease, diabetes and hypertension.

For many people the benefits of ablation will outweigh the risk, but it is important to discuss your individual risk factors with a knowledgeable and experienced practitioner.

A study has recently shown that patients who undergo ablation procedures reduce their stroke risk to that of the general population. Further studies are needed to find out whether indeed ablation is the reason for this whether external factors play a part or indeed whether the study was an anomaly. However, it's interesting to note that a similar effect occurs in patients with diabetes who undergo bariatric surgery. In many cases the diabetes spontaneously regresses directly after surgery and before lifestyle factors such as weight loss can occur. Maybe the human body possesses some hitherto undiscovered ability to heal itself when presented with a crisis such as the surgeon's knife or the ablator's catheter!

Modifiable Risk Factors for A-fib

Obesity and A-fib

Obesity has emerged as a major risk factor for the development of a-fib. Compared to healthy weight cohorts, obese individuals have up to a 2.4-fold increase in risk, and that risk increases as body mass index rises. The potential to progress from paroxysmal to permanent a-fib also increases with advancing weight. The good news is that weight loss not only reduces the frequency and length of a-fib episodes, it also reduces the potential for complications such as stroke and heart failure.

The effect of obesity on the cardiovascular system is profound. Related co-morbidities such as obstructive sleep apnoea and metabolic syndrome have already emerged as independent risk factors for the development of a-fib. Obesity can cause structural changes in the heart, increase atrial pressures, slow and disrupt conduction and cause a host of metabolic and haemo-dynamic changes which make a-fib far more amenable to induction. Obesity also causes vascular inflammation, another potent risk factor for a-fib.

The heart changes that occur in obesity can stretch the atria altering their electrical conduction. Over a decade obesity contributes to a 2.4-fold risk of left atrial enlargement visible on echo-cardiogram. Inflammation contributes to fibrosis and obesity alone is a risk factor for increased C-reactive protein levels, the marker for inflammation in the body.

A study in Australia looked at the hearts of sheep who had been intensively fed to induce obesity. The obese sheep demonstrated larger atrial volume and mass, slower atrial conduction, higher pressures in the left atrium, disordered atrial activity and a higher level of fibrotic markers when compared to non-obese sheep. Most tellingly, these sheep had a much higher susceptibility to both induced and spontaneous a-fib.

Similar findings in humans were demonstrated in a study carried out by the prestigious Mayo Clinic. In addition to increased atrial volume and pressure, the atria of obese humans had shorter refractory periods and slower conduction times.

Weight loss has been found to have a beneficial effect on reducing the burden of a-fib in many studies. In a presentation to the American Heart Association (Nov. 17, 2013) researchers revealed evidence that a weight loss of around 33 pounds could significantly reduce the frequency and length of a-fib episodes in obese patients. Patients who were put on a strict weight management plan experienced 2.5 times fewer episodes of a-fib and a 4.5 times reduction in symptoms.

Whether weight loss can reverse the structural and fibrotic changes in the heart that have already occurred is being studied. It is known that weight loss can reduce left ventricular hypertrophy, an enlargement of the ventricle often seen in obese subjects. Whether the same applies to the atria is not conclusively known although it is known that the progressive enlargement of the atria seen in obesity can be stopped by losing a large amount of weight (European Journal of Echocardiography. Sep 2008). Losing as little as 5% of body weight reduces levels of C-reactive protein and has shown to have a beneficial effect on the cardiovascular system.

Lastly, an encouraging story of a 51-year-old man scheduled for an ablation for persistent a-fib. The patient lost weight to reduce the complications of the surgery. After one month he spontaneously converted to sinus rhythm. Three months on and sinus rhythm persisted and the ablation was cancelled indefinitely.

A-Fib and Sleep Apnoea

Obstructive sleep apnoea is very strongly linked to atrial fibrillation, yet it is a condition which often goes undiagnosed. The correlation between the two conditions is so strong that many researchers now list OSA as a cause of a-fib rather than a co-existing condition. OSA can make a-fib resistant to anti-arrhythmic drugs, and its presence increases the risk of a-fib recurrence both after cardioversion and catheter ablation. It is really important then for a-fibbers to rule out OSA as a cause for their a-fib.

Obstructive sleep apnoea is a condition in which a person stops breathing for 10 seconds or more once an hour during sleep. As the throat relaxes, the soft tissues in the airway collapse and block or partially block the airways. The resultant drop in oxygen levels panics the brain into correcting the hypoxia by either rousing the sleeper or forcing them into a lighter level of sleep. This can happen hundreds of times per night, although the sleeper usually doesn't remember any of them. The result can be excess daytime sleepiness and irritability. Often OSA is linked with loud snoring, and as episodes of apnoea occur there may be gasping, choking and snorting. Many people with OSA have no clue there is a problem, unless their night time troubles are noticed by a partner or a friend. However, as OSA can lead to other problems, in addition to a-fib, it is really important to get it diagnosed and treated as soon as possible. Heavy snorers may like to consider having a sleep study done in order to rule out the condition.

The link between OSA and a-fib is very well established, with researchers estimating that at least 40% and perhaps 80% or more a-fibbers also have sleep apnoea. In one study, (Bitter T, Langer C, Vogt J, Horstkotte D, Oldenburg O 2009) OSA was present in 42.7% of those with a-fib. Another study

(Braga B, Poyares D, Cintra F et al 2009) found the number to be a shocking 81.6%. In the general population, about 5-10% of adults have some form of sleep apnoea, so the high levels observed in a-fibbers are truly remarkable. The relationship has also been found to be true in reverse. Someone with a diagnosis of OSA but no a-fib has a 4 times increased risk of developing the a-fib in the future.

So how does OSA cause a-fib? It is likely that a combination of factors are to blame. Firstly, dynamic and increasing intra-thoracic pressures may lead to structural changes in the heart including left atrial stretch (a significant marker for a-fib) and atrial remodelling. Hypoxia alters blood chemistry and activates the sympathetic nervous system releasing catecholamines. Negative tracheal pressures can also enhance vagal tone thus shortening atrial refractory periods.

The risk of developing OSA increases with rising body mass and can be reduced with weight loss. Obesity, OSA, hypertension and a-fib are commonly seen together with obesity the aggravating factor in many cases. Interestingly, OSA itself can cause weight gain, and once OSA is effectively controlled, it may be significantly easier to lose weight.

Diagnosis of OSA is done with a sleep study, either in a special sleep clinic or at home. The degree of OSA may be classed as none, mild, moderate or severe. Moderate to severe OSA is usually treated often with a device called CPAP (constant positive airway pressure). This is a mask which is worn during sleep and uses mild air pressure to hold the airways open. Mild OSA may be treatable by lifestyle changes such as weight loss and smoking cessation.

Untreated OSA can be a serious condition and eventually could even lead to a type of right sided heart failure called cor pulmonale. For the a-fib patient it could mean the different between a successful cardioversion or ablation and recurrence. Treatment with CPAP reduces the chance of post procedure recurrence almost back to baseline.

A-fib and Thyroid

Dysfunction of the thyroid gland is another modifiable cause of atrial fibrillation. A-fib usually affects people with an over-active thyroid or hyperthyroidism which is a condition which is 10 times more common in women than men. In an over-active thyroid, the body makes too much thyroxine causing the bodies functions to speed up. This results in symptoms such as palpitations, sweating, nervousness, trembling and irritability.

A-fib is present in 10-15% of people with an over-active thyroid gland and often resolves when the underlying condition is treated. Thyroid levels are often checked as a matter of course in all patients with new onset a-fib but this may not be routine. Thyroid dysfunction should certainly be considered especially in young women presenting with unexplained a-fib.

A-fib and Dental Disease

It is well established that bacteria in the mouth can impact the heart. Oral bacteria can enter the blood stream during dental or oral procedures where it can travel to the heart valves and cause endocarditis. This is why anti-biotic prophylaxis is usually offered to patients who have damaged heart valves, certain heart defects and cardiomyopathy, prior to any surgical procedure. However, infected root canals and other dental problems could also be contributing to low level inflammation which can aggravate a-fib. It is believed that chronic pockets of inflammation could increase levels of c-reactive protein indicating a systemic inflammatory response.

Some a-fibbers believe that mercury in amalgam fillings could be responsible for their episodes. Various theories have been put forward as to why this is including the fact that the metals in amalgam are capable of sustaining electrical currents in the mouth, or that there is a toxicity issue.   Unfortunately, there is little clear cut evidence to support amalgam removal. Amalgam removal requires a skilled practitioner who is experienced in minimizing exposure to mercury during the procedure.

Magnesium Deficiency and A-Fib

If you have a-fib you are most likely magnesium deficient. If you eat a typical diet, then you are probably magnesium deficient. If you have diabetes, metabolic syndrome or elevated blood sugar then you are almost certain to be magnesium deficient. An estimated 80% of the population are deficient in what has been called the miracle mineral. One of the signs of a magnesium deficiency? An erratic heartbeat.

Doctors have known for years that low levels of minerals can provoke arrhythmias even in healthy hearts. A small but very interesting study using post-menopausal women (J Am Coll Nutr. 2007 Apr;26(2):121-32.) found that even short periods of magnesium depletion i.e. a couple of months could induce heart rhythm changes in healthy people. Many of us have been deficient in magnesium for years! In the study, researchers aimed to assess whether restricting magnesium in the diet to about a third of the RDA would induce pathological changes. Magnesium in the diet would be restricted for 78 days and then repleted with 200mg of magnesium gluconate for a further 58 days. The results were startling. The heart rhythm changes induced in just under a third of the women before the 78 days was up meant that they had to enter the repletion part of the study early. 23% of the women in the study developed a-fib and aflutter. This responded well to magnesium repletion. In addition to inducing heart rhythm changes magnesium deficiency also increased the levels of glucose in blood serum and increased the levels of potassium and sodium in the urine. Elevated blood glucose levels can be induced by magnesium deficiency, which could address one of the other big epidemics of our time – diabetes.

Magnesium is responsible for over 300 functions in the body, yet the amount we get from diet alone has been steadily declining since the 1950's. The RDA for an adult is between

310mg and 420mg in the USA and in the UK it is 270-300mg. Studies show that the average adult has an intake far below the recommended level. It is not just our highly processed, sugar packed diets which are to blame, although sugar is a major depleter of magnesium. Between 1940 and 1991, the magnesium levels in vegetables dropped by 24% and in fruit by 16% due to mineral depletion in soil. Processing and cooking magnesium rich foods reduce the levels even more.

Magnesium deficiency is likely to be even more widespread than currently suspected due to the inefficacy of current tests. You may have previously been checked for magnesium deficiency and told your levels were fine. This is because the standard blood test for magnesium is a blood test and just 1% of the bodies total magnesium is contained in the blood. What is more the body makes an effort to maintain the amount in the blood at the expense of other parts of the body. So you could have been told that your magnesium levels were normal when in effect you were deficient in magnesium. Whilst there are other more expensive methods of testing for magnesium deficiency if you have any symptoms on the following list then you may want to increase your intake of magnesium and see if improvements occur.

Symptoms of a Magnesium Deficiency

Muscle twitching, spasms, tics
Irritability
Anxiety and panic attacks
Tiredness and lethargy
Inability to sleep
Inability to "Switch Off"
Seizures
Irregular or rapid heartbeat
Coronary spasms
Potassium deficiency
Impaired glucose tolerance
Hyperglycaemia
Tremors

Difficulty swallowing
Dizziness
Numbness and tingling
PMS
High blood pressure
Carb cravings
Craving for salt
Insomnia
Loss of appetite
Nausea
GERD
Confusion
Personality changes
Asthma and breathing difficulties
Chronic fatigue syndrome
ADHD
Tooth decay
Gum disease.

Magnesium Deficiency and Atrial Fibrillation

Magnesium plays a major role in the electrical function of the heart. It prolongs the atrial and atrioventricular refractory periods making the initiation of a-fib much less likely. Atrial tissue with inadequate magnesium is electrically unstable and irritable. By slowing atrial conduction times and increasing refractory periods, magnesium reduces potential arrhythmic events in the heart.

The idea that idiopathic arrhythmias are caused by nutritional/mineral deficiencies has been put forward by several experts in natural medicine including Dr Matthias Rath. One group who seem prone to idiopathic a-fib are athletes, particularly those who compete in endurance sports such as marathon running. This seeming paradox that the fittest elite are prone to cardiac arrhythmias has spawned several theories of why that may be. Whilst some doctors believe that the enlargement of the heart seen in athletic fitness could stretch the atria and make them more prone to fibrillate, it is also entirely feasible that these activities which are known to deplete electrolytes could result in long term mineral depletion. Endurance activities no doubt increase the bodies need for minerals substantially more than normal activities and it could be a long term subclinical deficit which is responsible for their arrhythmic episodes.

Many a-fibbers have testified to the success of magnesium in reducing or terminating their episodes and some have even cured the arrhythmia completely with magnesium alone. I am one of these lucky people. I now feel that my a-fib was the manifestation of a long standing mineral deficiency which in hindsight had caused problems for a while. Co-incidentally, in my youth I was also an endurance athlete – a swimmer which may or may not have contributed to my later problems. Prior to my first episode of a-fib I had experienced a very stressful year. It was my final year at university as a mature student and my thesis was due. I had stated to suffer panic attacks, to the point where I was unable to sit still in lectures and spent my final year studying alone in the library, ensuring I sat close to the door in case I needed to make an escape. I started to take a diet supplement which worked by absorbing dietary fat – and vitamins and minerals! Because of this I was advised to take a vitamin and mineral supplement, advice I did not heed.

The last two weeks of term involved the inevitable parties and social events, and although I was not a regular drinker I consumed a fair amount of alcohol, which no doubt depleted the last remaining minerals in my body. My diet was also appalling, usually junk food and full of refined sugar. I had started to experience reactive hypoglycaemia episodes where if I did not eat I would experience horrendous symptoms such as racing heart, sweating and shaking. So I gorged on refined sugar and processed food even more just to keep the horrible symptoms at bay. Finally, my body could take no more and "rewarded" me with my first episode of a-fib. The doctors at the hospital scratched their heads, they could find no reason for an apparently healthy young woman turning up in the emergency department with an arrhythmia which they said usually affected older people and people with heart disease. My magnesium levels were not checked at the hospital although they ran a battery of other tests and after three days I was released with a diagnosis of non-life threatening idiopathic atrial fibrillation cause unknown.

Two months later I arrived back in the emergency department, this time with a pulse of 160 bpm but regular. Three hours later when a doctor finally saw me I was rushed straight into resuscitation. Fearing I was about to expire, an adrenaline rush saw my pulse spike at 180 bpm. After a couple of pushes of adenosine which failed to do anything to slow my racing heart my pulse was still around 170. A consultant cardiologist was called and he diagnosed.... a panic attack! Slowly my pulse came down to 108 bpm and I was told to go away and stop worrying and maybe take a beta blocker to calm my nerves.

I now know that these were both manifestations of a very low magnesium level but it took me longer than I care to admit to figure it out. Over the few years, my heart continued to drop in and out of a-fib and I had interminable runs of ectopic beats, episodes of tachycardia and quite frankly my life became a living hell. Unless you have a-fib it is nearly impossible to understand the havoc it can wreak on your quality of life. It is always there in the back of your mind, wondering whether today will be the day you end up in the emergency room or when it will strike. I had been studying with the intention of becoming a primary school teacher but that plan fell by the wayside. I became very withdrawn and lost my independence, scared to even go out on my own because of the fear of an attack in a public place.

One particular night I was lay on the sofa trying to watch a film with my heart seemingly skipping every other beat. "I've had enough of this I want answers", I said to my partner, who whilst supportive didn't understand what I was getting so worked up about. His attitude was its not going to kill you so why worry, oh if only it was that simple! Luckily providence was on my side that night as I consulted Dr Google because the very first result I found was a lady who had cured her skipped heartbeat problem by using magnesium supplements.

The next day with my heart still skipping madly I rushed out to the shop and purchased some chelated magnesium. This was my second piece of luck. At that point I didn't understand the different types of magnesium or their bio-availability so the fact that I picked chelated was pure chance. If ever there was evidence that magnesium deficiency was the root of my problems, then this was it. Within a couple of hours my skipped beats had subsided considerably and within a day or two they were completely gone. I rushed to tell my doctor my miracle cure but she was most unimpressed. There is no link between arrhythmia and magnesium she said... Unfortunately, I found out this was not an uncommon phenomenon with the medical profession. Doctors often dismiss non pharmaceutical interventions or natural remedies offhand, even when patients present clear evidence that it is working for them.

However, I was not out of the woods yet even though my heart was rock solid and steady. I got sloppy with taking the magnesium. I ran out and didn't bother to replace them. After all, I had experienced no more a-fib, no more ectopic beats I was cured wasn't I? A couple of months later I experienced a very traumatic event. My daughter ended up in hospital after an accident and she had lost a lot of blood. It was touch and go but happily she pulled through and made a full recovery. Nevertheless, two weeks later I felt the familiar flip flop and bang into a-fib for five hours. Stress is a major depleter of magnesium and I had been under intense mental and physical stress. I hadn't eaten properly, I had worried for days and had stopped the magnesium. I picked up my magnesium routine in earnest, switching this time to magnesium citrate powder and once again my heart settled into its normal steady beat. I was to experience only a couple more a-fib events after that and they were definitely linked to magnesium deficiency. One was during a particularly nasty sickness and diarrhoea bug when I had vomited for three days solid and could not keep anything down. This one converted within minutes of forcing down magnesium and potassium. The other was again when I was slack with my minerals and under stress.

Since then I have experienced no more episodes of a-fib, I occasionally get atrial ectopic beats which I take as a sign I need to up my magnesium intake. It always works. I now consider myself cured so long as I maintain magnesium at a reasonable level. I read my body for signs I am getting low – eyelid and muscle twitches, ectopic beats and up my intake if necessary. I take no medication and have not seem my doctor for arrhythmia for over 5 years. For me magnesium has been a miracle.

Resolving Magnesium Deficiency.

Just as it can take months to years for a mineral deficiency to arise, so it can take months to years to correct it. Some people try magnesium supplementation for a short time and declare it doesn't work for them. Some people are using the wrong supplements entirely, certain forms of magnesium are next to useless when it comes to resolving a deficiency. It is a paradox but once the body becomes very low in magnesium it becomes increasingly hard to correct it. Magnesium deficient subjects may have great difficulty absorbing certain types of magnesium or indeed any at all. If your magnesium level is low, your potassium level may be low too as the two need each other for absorption. Before using any form of supplement, particularly potassium please check with and get the consent of your doctor. Magnesium is generally considered very safe in people with normal kidney function but nevertheless ask the advice of your doctor or health care provider before proceeding.

Magnesium Rich Foods
The following foods are good natural sources of magnesium and should be incorporated into your diet as much possible.

Pumpkin Seeds
Spinach
Swiss Chard
Yoghurt/Kefir
Almonds
Black Beans
Avocado
Figs
Dark Chocolate
Banana
Salmon
Nuts and Seeds
Coriander
Coffee – not great for many a-fibbers
Kelp
Rice Bran

Magnesium Supplementation
Most people with a magnesium deficiency will need to use some form of supplement. However not all supplements are equal or effective. Magnesium oxide which is the most common and inexpensive form of magnesium found in supplements is very poorly absorbed with around 4% of standard supplements actually being available to the body. Therefore, a 500mg tablet will provide just 12mg of magnesium.

Better forms of magnesium include magnesium glycinate, magnesium taurate and magnesium citrate.

Magnesium glycinate is a chelated form of magnesium, which means it is bound to an amino acid, in this case glycine which increases its bio availability in the body. Magnesium glycinate is also less likely to cause loose stools than other forms of magnesium. Approximately 80% of magnesium glycinate is absorbed.

Magnesium taurate is a compound of magnesium and taurine

which is an amino acid. Taurine possesses anti-arrhythmic properties, decreases irritability of heart tissues and helps to regulate magnesium, sodium and potassium levels within cells. It is considered a helpful supplement by many people with a-fib and is sometimes used together with arginine to reduce the frequency of ectopic beats – both PVC's and PAC's.

Magnesium citrate is a readily available, cheap and well absorbed form of magnesium but unfortunately it does have laxative effects in higher doses – so much so that it is actually marketed as a laxative. Magnesium citrate is available in powder form as well as capsules so you can experiment with a dose which doesn't cause bowel problems. Magnesium citrate is excreted quite quickly by your body so it is recommended it is used several times per day in small doses.

Magnesium malate is a form of magnesium which is found helpful by a-fibbers and sufferers of fibromyalgia and chronic fatigue syndrome alike. Malic acid helps to increase energy production and some studies have found it useful in reducing blood pressure although there is not yet enough evidence to consider using it for this purpose alone.

All forms of oral magnesium can have laxative effects although this is more likely with some forms than others. Diarrhoea is counterproductive as it leaches even more magnesium and also potassium from your body which can worsen a deficiency. If you experience loose bowels cut back on oral magnesium and consider using transdermal magnesium which is another highly bio-available form of magnesium.

Transdermal Magnesium
Transdermal magnesium is a topical form of magnesium chloride which is very easily absorbed and highly effective in treating aches and pains, sports injuries and repleting magnesium stores.   This ancient form of the mineral comes from ancient sea beds such as the Zechstein sea bed in

Northern Europe where it is naturally protected from modern pollutants. The magnesium is then ionized to allow it to be absorbed through the skin. As the skin is the largest organ in the body absorption occurs quickly, and the convenience of this form of magnesium allows it to be applied directly to any part of the body.

Transdermal magnesium comes in several forms, the most popular of which is an "oil" spray which is not really an oil at all but a solution of approximately 31% of magnesium chloride in purified water. Transdermal magnesium products also include lotions, gels, balms, foot soaks and bath flakes which can be added to the tub for a relaxing and repleting soak.

Transdermal magnesium can replete body stores approximately five times faster than oral supplementation and has none of the laxative side effects. It is therefore safe to use on children (use small amounts on children under 12) and during pregnancy. Dosage varies by the manufacturer but looking at two magnesium oil products I have here on my desk, 10 sprays of one provides 150mg and the other 180mg providing 43% and 60% of the UK RDA respectively.

Magnesium chloride flakes can be added to baths or used as a foot-bath. For a bath dissolve around 250mg (UK measure) of flakes in a bath of warm water and soak for around 20 minutes. In a foot-bath use around 150mg. Repeat 2-3 times per week for optimal efficiency.

Whilst magnesium oils are not expensive, beware of very cheap magnesium products which may be magnesium sulphate (Epsom Salts). Whilst Epsom Salts can be used trans dermally (see below) they are not as effective or well absorbed as magnesium chloride. Top quality oils use a solution of 31% Zechstein magnesium with 100 ml providing around 800 sprays.

Correcting a minor magnesium deficiency with transdermal magnesium takes around 4 – 6 weeks, much faster than oral magnesium supplementation which takes an average 6 months. Side effects are rare but it may cause tingling and local irritation on application to start with, particularly if you are very low on magnesium. If you are using it on broken skin you may need to dilute the solution to around 4% as it will sting!

If you have little success with oral magnesium, consider transdermal magnesium before giving up on it altogether. If you have previously used magnesium oxide it is very unlikely that this will have had much effect if any on your a-fib. Try a month of transdermal therapy and see the difference it makes.

Epsom Salts – Magnesium Sulphate

Magnesium sulphate is one of the major components of bath salts, as it is very inexpensive. It is also used medically in IV drips used in cardiac arrest, for correcting the ventricular arrhythmia Torsades de Pointes, and in asthma as a bronchodilator. Used orally it is a very potent laxative.

Used trans dermally magnesium sulphate has some success in raising magnesium levels but not nearly as successfully as magnesium chloride. One British study found that a 1% solution of Epsom Salts – 600 grams in a 15 US gallon tub raised body magnesium levels mildly in most of the subjects tested. There were no adverse effects. The optimal amount to use is 500-600grams in a standard bath at 40 degrees and soak for 12 minutes according to the study.

Epsom Salts are not recommended for use orally for repleting magnesium due to the extreme laxative effect!

Magnesium Overdose

Magnesium overdose is very rare in people with normal kidney function as healthy kidneys will filter out the excess. Nevertheless, magnesium overdose could be an issue with renal impairment or when mega amounts of the mineral are ingested. This is why it is important to check that it is safe to take magnesium with your health care provider prior to supplementation.

<u>Signs of a Magnesium overdose</u>
Low blood pressure
Slow breathing
Slow heart rate and or erratic heart rhythm
Shortness of breath
Dizziness
In very severe cases cardiac arrest

If you or someone else has consumed very large doses of magnesium and the above signs appear seek immediate medical care.

Low Potassium Levels in A-fib

Low potassium levels are another potent trigger for arrhythmias and anyone with a-fib should have their levels of potassium checked if it has not been done already. Normal blood levels of potassium are 3.5 – 5 mmo/L with levels below 3.5 mmo/L considered low. Potassium is very important to the heart, and a severe deficiency can cause cardiac arrest. All muscles, and of course the heart is a big muscle need potassium in order to contract correctly. The differing levels of potassium in the cells (intracellular) and outside of the cells (extracellular) drives the contraction process. When levels of potassium in the body drop low the normally distinct balance between intracellular and intracellular decrease and muscles become twitchy and excitable and in the case of the heart prone to arrhythmia.

Because potassium is so important to heart function, it is common to test potassium levels in the emergency room when presenting with certain cardiac conditions, particularly arrhythmia. Potassium is generally quite abundant in the diet so major dietary deficiencies are quite rare, however certain medications such as diuretics are known for depleting potassium stores. This is why doctors often prescribe supplements when prescribing these drugs. Other causes of low potassium include dehydration, particularly after prolonged diarrhoea or vomiting, eating disorders, alcoholism and bariatric surgery.

Symptoms of low potassium include weakness, numbness and tingling, tiredness, palpitations, stomach pain and bloating, constipation, paralysis, frequent urination, increased thirst, low blood pressure, abnormal heart rhythms, fainting and depression.

Repletion of potassium using supplements should be done under medical supervision as too much can be as harmful as too little. People taking ACE inhibitors are usually instructed to avoid potassium supplements and people with kidney disease may need to avoid both supplements and high potassium foods such as bananas, oranges, tomatoes, peaches and cantaloupe melon.

Magnesium deficiency can worsen a potassium deficiency as the two need each other in order to be absorbed efficiently. In fact, if an underlying magnesium deficiency is present, it is very hard to correct a potassium deficiency. Magnesium is often administered at the same time as potassium for this reason.

Vitamins and Minerals Which May Be Beneficial For A-Fib

<u>Vitamin C</u>

Vitamin C has proved to be very beneficial in preventing the post-operative a-fib which often follows cardiac surgery. It is believed to occur in up to 40% of procedures. A small yet impressive study by Eslami et al found that giving 2000mg of vitamin C prior to surgery and 1000mg twice a day for a further five days afterwards could reduce the incidence of post-operative a-fib by 85%. Vitamin C also appears to be effective in the prevention of recurrence after a successful cardioversion for a-fib. In one study, supplementation with Vitamin C before and for a week after cardioversion led to recurrence in just 4.5% of Vitamin C treated patients as opposed to over 36% of patients in a control group.

Vitamin C has long been considered a queller of inflammation in the body and it is in this capacity that its most likely to be useful in a-fib. Vitamin C has the capacity to lower levels of C-reactive protein in individuals with raised levels, reduce oxidative stress and lower other markers of inflammation which could play a role in initiating attacks,

The current RDA of 75-90mg has been suggested to be woefully low by supporters of vitamin C therapy, who argue that smokers, people with chronic illness particularly cardiovascular disease need much higher levels. Vitamin c has a relatively low toxicity and excess levels are excreted from the body. The US food and nutrition board set a tolerable upper intake level of 2000mg for adults, mainly to prevent gastrointestinal upset and diarrhoea which results from excessive intake.

If you are taking blood thinners like Warfarin, be aware that high doses of Vitamin C may decrease the effectiveness of the drug. Regular supplementation may require a higher dose of Warfarin so be sure to talk this over with your doctor and ensure your INR levels are checked regularly.

Taurine

Taurine is an amino acid which plays many roles in the function of a healthy body, but is particularly abundant in the heart. It is often considered a "heart beat regulator" due to its ability to calm irritable heart tissue, improve contraction and dampen sympathetic nervous system activity. It's role in eradicating arrhythmia has been the subject of several studies, most notably one by George Eby and William Halcomb who found that taurine in combination with another amino acid l'arginine was very successful in eliminating premature heart beats (PVC's and PAC's) and a-fib. The study hypothesized that cardiac arrhythmias occurring in otherwise healthy people could be due to deficiencies of taurine and l'arginine.

Taurine occurs naturally in some foods, most notably in meat and fish. The body can also manufacture it so long as there is adequate intake of vitamin B6. The demand for taurine may outweigh its supply particularly as the body ages, during periods of chronic illness or stress, in abnormal glucose states such as diabetes and when taurine is restricted in the diet i.e. vegan and some vegetarian diets. Chemicals in food may also reduce taurine levels in the body – monosodium glutamate (MSG) and aspartame are two such culprits, and interesting both of these substances are listed as potential dietary a-fib triggers. Perhaps these substances contribute to an underlying taurine deficiency?

Taurine is essential for a multitude of different processes in the body. In the heart it moves sodium and potassium in and out of cells and aids electrical stabilization. It can relieve arrhythmia, angina, high blood pressure and prevents cardiomyopathy. It is also essential for repairing damage in the retina of the eye, it enhances the immune system, moderates blood sugar levels, is useful in the prevention and treatment of liver diseases, protects against ageing – the list is almost endless. In animal studies Taurine has been shown to reduce the risk of dying from heart failure by nearly 80%. Taurine has also been linked with longevity, studies have shown that the residents of Japan who have the longest life expectancies also have a diet that is high in taurine.

Fish Oils

Results from studies into the efficacy of fish oil for preventing a-fib and other arrhythmias have been mixed. Whilst fish oil has been proven to be effective in the prevention and treatment of several cardiovascular disorders and many other diseases, its role in the prevention or management of a-fib has never been conclusively proven. Finnish researchers (Virtanen, JK, et al) did find evidence that high blood levels of DHA (one of the components of fish oil) to be associated with a 49% reduced risk of atrial fibrillation. However, another study (Nigam et al) found fish oil to be of no benefit to a-fibbers.

Further studies have been done looking at the two major components in fish oil – DHA and EPA. In one dog study. (Ramadeen et al) found that a-fib conductibility was significant decreased in the group being given DHA and atrial fibrosis improved

In contrast, a Japanese study (Tomita et al) found that EPA levels were higher in a-fib patients than in controls and that EPA may even be a precipitating factor for AF.

This research is very confusing for a-fibbers, but it seems that pure DHA fish oil is preferable to EPA, if you choose to use fish oils at all.

Vitamin D

Vitamin D deficiency has been suggested as a possible factor for non-valvular a-fib (Demir et al). Their study found that vitamin D levels were lowest in patients with non-valvular AF when compared to patients with mitral valve disease and healthy patients. Other studies however have found whilst there is a correlation between very low levels of Vitamin D and other forms of cardiovascular disease such as CAD and heart failure, these findings do not apply to AF. To complicate matters even further, at a meeting of The American Heart Association evidence was presented that excess Vitamin D significantly increases the risk of atrial fibrillation. So what are we supposed to believe?

In fairness, the study used at the AHA presentation did find that only patients with very high levels of Vitamin D (100 ng/ml and higher) were at 2.5 times greater risk of developing A-fib. These are excessive levels and reasonably hard to achieve. The study didn't find any increased risk with lower levels but they did agree that Vitamin D deficiency was associate with an increased risk of hypertension, diabetes and heart failure.

Whether or not Vitamin D supplementation is useful in a-fib is still unclear.

Diet and A-Fib

Dietary triggers for a-fib can be diverse and it can be very challenging to establish what foods are causing you problems. If you have a known food allergy, then it is important to eliminate those foods from your diet completely to minimise the inflammatory reaction which can worsen a-fib. However, many dietary triggers are much more subtle and it can take some intensive detective work to figure them out. It helps to keep a diary of all the foods and drink you consume so you can work out if diet is the culprit for your episodes.

MSG Monosodium Glutamate

MSG is well recognised for causing sensitivity in some people, so much so that the phenomena has even been given a name Chinese Restaurant Syndrome. Glutamate can cause problems by competing with cysteine, an amino acid which is essential for the production of taurine, an important amino acid for maintaining a regular heartbeat. Symptoms of MSG sensitivity usually start within 2 hours of consuming food containing it and include irregular and erratic heartbeat, racing heart, skipped beats, headache, flushing, nausea and sweating, numbness and burning in the mouth. For some people the reaction can be so intense that they think they are having a heart attack.

MSG also known as E621 and Vetsin is used as a flavour enhancer and is commonly used in Asian cooking and processed foods, especially crisps (chips), chicken and sausage products, sauces and dressings, and ready meals. Although many food manufacturers have made an effort to reduce or eliminate MSG in their products a stroll through any grocery stores snack aisles shows that it is still very prevalent in the foods available. In a study carried out by the excellent

A-fib Report, 10% of respondents lists MSG as a trigger for their attacks.

One of the most compelling pieces of evidence that MSG can trigger a-fib comes from the International Journal of Cardiology (Feb 9, 2009). The patient was a 57-year-old physician who was being treated for paroxysmal a-fib and considering catheter ablation. He then cut out all MSG and aspartame (another potential a-fib trigger) from his diet and his a-fib stopped completely. To test that it was indeed these substances that were triggering his a-fib, he set himself three separate challenges – two with MSG and one with aspartame. Each time he consumed foods containing the substances he went into a-fib within hours.

Free glutamate by contrast is a naturally occurring substance in many foods and is often considered beneficial to health, but some evidence finds that even that can cause sensitivity in some people. Foods high in natural glutamate include Parmesan and aged cheeses, soy sauce, fish sauce, mushrooms, ripe tomatoes, grape juice, gluten, malt barley, beef jerky, pork, chicken and potatoes. So if your pizza is sending you into a-fib, you could have a sensitivity to free glutamate.

Tyramine
Tyramine is a compound which occurs natural in certain foods particularly aged and fermented cheeses, fish and meat. It is also found in yoghurt, soy sauce, sour cream, sauerkraut, sour dough breads, yeast extract and over ripe and dried fruit. Tyramine can also be found in wine, particularly red wine. Ingestion of tyramine can trigger a-fib attacks in some individuals. Aged cheese and red wine seem to be particularly potent triggers for initiating an attack. Tyramine rich foods should be avoided by patients taking MAO inhibitors as they can cause dangerously high blood pressure reactions.

Aspartame
Aspartame or E951 is an artificial sweetener which is used in

an increasing number of sweetened foods and drinks. One research study by Dr H J Roberts found that 16% of those listed in his database as aspartame reactors named arrhythmia as one of the effects of consumption. Another study by The A-fib Report found that 4% of a-fibbers listed aspartame as a trigger. products, many of which are labelled as low calories, low sugar or sugar free. Products in which aspartame is found include diet soda, desserts, toppings, shakes, beverage sweeteners and even some vitamins and toothpaste. Whilst aspartame doesn't cause problems for many people it seems it is capable of initiating a-fib episodes as we saw in the earlier experiment described in this chapter,

Caffeine
Many people with a-fib avoid caffeine and another stimulants as a matter of course. However recent studies show that caffeine may not be as bad for a-fib sufferers as previously thought. A study in the American Journal of Clinical Nutrition found that moderate caffeine use had no effect on atrial arrhythmias and there was no clinical benefit to abstinence. One study published in the Canadian Journey of Cardiology found that caffeine may even lower incidence of a-fib This intriguing finding revealed a 6% relative risk reduction in incidence of a-fib for every 300g per day habitually drunk! Whilst caution is urged in the interpretation of the study, one speculation is that caffeine may actually have an anti-fibrotic effect on the atria, thus protecting against a-fib. The good news for a-fibbers is that you probably can have that morning coffee without worrying about it

Alcohol
Excessive alcohol consumption is known to trigger a-fib even in people with no history of the condition – the so called Holiday Heart Syndrome. It is not clear exactly why alcohol can cause a-fib but it is a well-known fact in emergency rooms around the world that during holidays and other celebrations, admissions for a-fib soar. Binge drinking, overindulgence and stress cause a host of transient arrhythmias in normal healthy subjects and fall under the umbrella of Holiday Heart. The

exact mechanism of alcohol induced arrhythmia has not been identified but various theories such as dehydration, adrenaline release and mineral depletion have been postulated. Magnesium in particular is depleted by alcohol, so Holiday Heart could be the result of a borderline magnesium deficiency. In most cases, the heart rhythm returns to normal on its own and no further treatment is needed other than avoiding excess alcohol.

Whilst binge drinking is clearly a risk factor for a-fib, what about moderate or light drinking? A recent study in Sweden using a population without a-fib set out to examine how much various levels of alcohol consumption increased the risk of a-fib. Three levels of alcohol consumption: 1-6 drinks per week, 7-14 drinks per week and 14 plus drinks per week were studied. The study also looked at the type of alcohol consumed, wine, spirits and beer.
The fact that the study found any degree of alcohol consumption increased risk of a-fib wasn't unexpected. However, the level of risk and the type of alcohol drank was quite surprising. A single glass of wine per day raised risk by just 2%. However, when consumption increased to two glasses of wine per day the risk jumped to 35%. Low levels of spirit consumption - 1-6 drinks per week increased risk by 5% whereas 14 drink or more a week increased the risk by 46%. However, the oddest set of results come with beer consumption. 1-6 drinks per week did not raise risk at all, 7-14 drinks raised risk by 11% but with 14 or more drinks per week the risk dropped back down to 3%.

Everyone is different with a varying tolerance to alcohol. Some of the effects of drinking on a-fib could probably be offset by avoiding dehydration and ensuring mineral levels are optimised. Avoiding alcohol entirely is not a practical or enjoyable prospect for many of us although it is no doubt what many doctors would recommend!

Wheat and Gluten
Dramatic improvements in a-fib have been reported by some

patients after the adoption of a wheat and gluten free diet. Research has shown that the risk of a-fib is slighter higher in individuals with Coeliac disease (extreme sensitivity to gluten) than in the general population. About 1-2% of the population have Coeliac disease, yet around 30% of people carry genetic markers for the disease. Around 80 % of people with coeliac disease are undiagnosed.

Symptoms of coeliac disease include diarrhoea, cramping, bloating, weight loss, lethargy and vomiting, plus a host of seemingly unrelated complications including skin rashes and epilepsy.

Ingesting wheat and gluten can cause inflammation in the bodies of sensitive individuals and it is this inflammation which is thought to contribute to the initiation of a-fib. The link between a-fib and inflammation has been well established by many studies, with patients with a-fib consistently having higher levels of C-reactive protein, a marker for systemic inflammation than those in normal sinus rhythm. Those with persistent a-fib have higher levels of CRP than those with paroxysmal a-fib leading to the hypothesis that a-fib is the result of some form of inflammatory process in the body.

It is important to note that intolerance and allergy are not the same thing. Allergies involve an auto immune response and the body produces antibodies in response to the perceived threat to the body. Allergies can be diagnosed with a blood test. Intolerances do not provoke an immune response but exposure brings on symptoms, which may vary with the length and type of exposure. Diagnosing wheat intolerance requires a food challenge under controlled conditions.

Coeliac disease diagnosis begins with a blood test for antibodies. If antibodies are found, a biopsy of the gut can confirm the disease.

For anyone wanting to lower or eliminate their intake of wheat and gluten the Paleo diet has provided successful for several a-fib patients including some who were able to eliminate the disorder altogether using diet alone. The Paleo diet is described as a hunter gatherer diet and places high emphasis on meat and protein, high fibre and non-starchy fruits and vegetables. Grains including wheat, dairy products, refined sugar, salt, legumes and alcohol are eliminated from the Paleo diet.

Salt

Excessive salt consumption can be a problem for people with a-fib. Not only is salt suspected of raising blood pressure in sensitive individuals by causing the body to retain fluid but it also depletes magnesium and potassium in the body – minerals essential for retaining a healthy heartbeat. Looking back at the diary I kept during my episodes, many of them started after eating foods high in salt. Potassium and sodium are both electrolytes which the body must retain in balance in order to function correctly. If too much of one is consumed, the other will be released by the body to maintain balance. Therefore, eating too much salt will cause the body to leech potassium. The average diet is rarely deficient in sodium as it occurs naturally in many foods but potassium is a problem for some a-fibbers. There are various salt substitutes on the market which use potassium chloride rather than sodium chloride which is the prime ingredient in regular table salt. If you think that salt may be contributing to your a-fib attacks it may be worth switching to one of these, but discuss it with your doctor first. Potassium based salt substitutes can be dangerous in people with renal impairment who need to watch their potassium intake. Another option is pure sea salt which retains some of the mineral content which is removed from table salt.

Dairy Products

Occasionally anecdotal evidence pops up to suggest that eliminating dairy products from the diet has helped or even eliminated a-fib. Although I have researched and tried to find clinical evidence to support this theory, so far all I have found is word of mouth accounts. I am not doubting the veracity of these accounts – after all a cure is a cure however it is achieved but hard clinical data is definitely lacking on this one. The only possible conclusion I can draw from these account is that either the individuals concerned had an underlying lactose intolerance which was contributing to inflammation in their bodies or their a-fib stemmed from excessive calcium intake which excites the heart. Calcium however is an essential component of a healthy heart, it helps with contraction and nerve conduction, besides being necessary for strong bones and teeth. The best form of it is in dairy products. Low calcium levels prolong the QT interval in the heart which increases the risk of serious ventricular arrhythmia. Proceed with caution.

Sugar
Sugar can be a trigger for a-fib attacks and indeed a-fib is associated with high blood sugar states such as diabetes and impaired glucose tolerance. The famous Framingham heart study found diabetes to be an independent risk factor for a-fib in the early 1990's, and since then numerous studies have been carried out which link higher blood glucose states with the development of a-fib. In one Japanese study, diabetes increased the risk of women developing a-fib by 26%. As the body's glucose mechanisms begin to falter, insulin levels start to rise and with increased level of insulin comes increased production of arachidonic acid. This helps to build eicosanoids which help to increase inflammation in the body. Not only that but high insulin levels kick starts the production of interleukin 6, which creates C-reactive protein, the marker for inflammation which is higher in people with a-fib.

Even in people with normal blood glucose and other high glycaemic foods have the potential to cause inflammation in the body. Sugar depletes important minerals such as magnesium which explains why people who live on high carb, high sugar diets almost always have low magnesium levels. If that wasn't bad enough, research published in the Journal of American Medicine found that higher levels of sugar in the diet increased the risk of dying from cardiovascular causes considerably. Those who got around a fifth of their daily calories from sugar increased their risk of dying from heart attack or stroke by 28% compared to those who got just 8% of their daily calories from sugar.

The Connection Between A-fib and H-Pylori.

H-pylori is a bacterium which lives in the gut and affects around 50% of the world's population. For most people it doesn't cause a problem, yet in some people h-pylori causes a chronic inflammation of the stomach lining leading to gastritis and ulcers. In fact, over 90% of ulcer disease is caused by this insidious bacterium.

An interesting study publish in Heart in June 2005 documented that not only did a high percentage of people who presented in the cardiology department have gastric problems, but also that a significant marker of systemic inflammation – CRP or C Reactive Protein was much higher in a-fib patients than in the general population. In fact, a-fib patients were 20 times more likely to test positive for h-pylori than healthy volunteers and their CRP levels were 5 times as high!

It has often been suggested that a-fib in the absence of structural heart disease could be caused by some kind of inflammatory process going on in the body. Whilst the link between a-fib and h-pylori has not been conclusively proved by large studies, there is a lot of anecdotal evidence from both patients and practitioners that treating h-pylori reduced a-fib events and even eliminated it entirely in some patients.

Unfortunately, h-pylori is a cunning little bug, designed to exist in the harshest acidic conditions in the stomach. It does this by burrowing into the cells which line the gut, where it provokes an inflammatory response. Unless the host develops symptoms such as bloating, upper abdominal discomfort, nausea, vomiting or signs of bleeding in the gastrointestinal tract, they are unlikely to know they have been infected. Most people with h-pylori never develop symptoms and unless h-pylori is actively eliminated, it can remain in the body indefinitely.

If you have a-fib and gastric symptoms or even if you have a-fib with no gastric symptoms, it is worth checking your h-pylori status.

Testing for H-Pylori.

There are three main methods to test for H-pylori.

Blood Tests
Antibodies to h-pylori can be detected in the blood and are most commonly used in people who have never been treated for the bug. This is because antibodies can remain in the blood for up to 18 months after H Pylori has been eliminated, so it is not a useful test to determine whether there is a current infection. What a blood test can tell you is whether you have been infected with H-Pylori in the past. If you test positive and have never been treated, it is likely that you still have a current infection. You can purchase a simple h-pylori home test kit at many pharmacies and online, or you can have the test carried out in your doctor's office.

Urea Breath Test
A urea breath test can be used to determine whether or not there is a current h-pylori infection and whether or not treatment has been successful. However, this test is quite expensive and is not routinely used. Also if you have taken antibiotics or used proton pump inhibitors or H2 receptor agonist drugs prior to the test it may not be accurate.

Stool Antigen Test
This is the most accurate way of determining current h-pylori status. A pea sized sample of stool is taken to check for antibodies. Again you should not have taken PPI or H2

receptor agonist drugs for at least two weeks prior to the test or antibiotics for four weeks.

Treating H Pylori

The most common treatment for h-pylori is a week-long triple combination therapy, consisting of two different types of antibiotics plus a proton pump inhibitor. Usually the antibiotics are a combination of either Amoxicillin and Clarithromycin or Metronidazole and Clarithromycin plus Omeprazole.

This combination of drugs is quite rough on the system but eliminates the infection about 85% of the time. If the initial treatment is unsuccessful it may be repeated using a different combination of drugs.

One alternative treatment which has proved quite useful in eradicating H pylori naturally is Mastic Gum. Mastic is a resin obtained from Pistacia Lentiscus, a tree native to the Mediterranean region. It has been used as a stomach tonic for centuries however recently it has been found to be able to suppress and even kill h-pylori.   The usual dose is 1g per day or four 250mg capsules taken just before bed. Mastic is not associated with any of the side effects of antibiotic therapy and has a low toxicity potential. Unfortunately, objective medical studies on how effective Mastic Gum is at clearing h-pylori are quite limited, although a study published in the New England Journal of Medicine (Dec 24 1998) found that Mastic had quite definite antibacterial activity against h pylori.

A second study (Dabos KJ1, Sfika E, Vlatta LJ, Giannikopoulos G.) found that Mastic alone eradicated H-Pylori in 30% and 38% respectively of the groups studied in only 14 days. Mastic therefore is a potential alternative treatment for those who cannot or do not want to take conventional triple combination therapy.

The Emotional Burden of A-fib and How to Overcome it.

Very little has been written about the emotional impact that a diagnosis of a-fib can bring. Certainly when I was first diagnosed I felt very isolated and alone, wondering how one day I was a healthy young woman and next day a patient in a cardiac ward. I wondered if I would ever get my life back, ever begin to feel normal, when the fear and pulse holding (I was a world expert at secretly taking my pulse) would end. Luckily, I have a friend who believes in tough love and after bemoaning to him the huge impact that a-fib was having on my life he uttered these golden words of advice. "A-fib can only ruin your life if you let it".

Whilst a-fib can be frightening, it is not generally considered a life threatening condition. The health risks which accompany it can be effectively managed. People even in permanent a-fib lead long, active and productive lives. When we feel overwhelmed by the condition, and I often did in those early days, it is worth focussing on these positives. The advances made over the past twenty years or so have transformed the landscape of a-fib which once seemed so barren and bare. More and more people are now free of the condition and a cure is on the horizon for many more. Above all with this condition there is hope, hope for a permanent and lasting cure.

It is probably the unpredictability of the disorder that has the biggest impact. A friend of mine once described paroxysmal a-fib as like a stalker, ready to pounce when you least expect it, whether it be in the middle of a family celebration or when you are trying to drift off to sleep at night. In the early days, my biggest fear was being carted off to hospital, as since my diagnosis I had developed a pathological fear of doctors and hospitals. I later found that I could deal with my episodes at home and that went a long way to easing my anxiety. Still, the

Nuisance as I called it was never far from my mind. It impacted my life in more ways than I care to admit. I had always prided myself on my independence yet almost overnight I became scared to leave the house alone. I abandoned my studies, I could not see how I could sit still in lectures when I feared my heart was about to leap out of my chest and explode. I gave up my ambition of becoming a primary school teacher, as I could imagine myself dashing out of the classroom in panic if an episode began! I sank into a deep depression.

Depression is common amongst many sufferers of chronic diseases, and a-fib is no exception. Thrall et al found that 38% of patients with a-fib had significant depression and approximately the same number displayed symptoms of anxiety. Women were particularly affected. If you are suffering from depression or anxiety as a result of your a-fib, I urge you to seek help as soon as possible.   There is so much that can be done to improve your quality of life, and for me this was the pivotal point in my quest to conquer a-fib. A short course of anti-depressants together with some CBT counselling helped me to put everything back into perspective and the strength to get determined to conquer this beast.

Another friend who fought an ongoing battle with a-fib attributed much of their anxiety to fear of the unknown. Doctors in general practice encounter a-fib so frequently it becomes a routine diagnosis much like the flu or acid reflux. Because of this they fail to fully explain the condition to patients and this can lead to a lot of unnecessary anxiety and fear. With a-fib education is the key to empowerment and the first step to conquering it. Become knowledgeable about the condition and much of the fear will melt away. It can help to make contact with others who are on the road to curing their a-fib for support. Your doctor may be able to put you in touch with local support groups and there are many online forums and groups that may be helpful too. Ensure too that you have the best medical support network, doctors who are knowledgeable, open minded and willing to involve you in decisions about your care. If you are going to fight a battle, you need the very best army around you

To return to the advice given by Mr Tough Love - "A-fib can only ruin your life if you let it", it's pretty blunt but it's true. You may not be able to control when a-fib strikes but you can control your reaction to it. A-fib can be conquered and it can be beaten but the important part is remaining positive.

Alternative Therapies

Yoga and A-fib

Yoga has been found to reduce the burden of a-fib and have a beneficial effect on mental health according to a study carried out by the University of Kansas Medical Center. The study followed a group of patients with paroxysmal atrial fibrillation for a period of six months. The initial part of the study, the control period followed the group going about their normal daily life for three months.

During the second three-month period, the group participated in a 1 hour Iyengar yoga class twice a week. The yoga classes consisted of 10 minutes of warm up exercises, 10 minutes of pranayamas, 30 minutes of asanas and 10 minutes of relaxation. The participants were also encouraged to practice yoga exercises daily at home.

During the yoga period of the study, a-fib burden dropped by 35-40% and 22% of the participants had no a-fib episodes at all. Mental health was positively impacted as was heart rate and blood pressure.

It is becoming increasingly clear that there is a strong connection to the autonomic nervous system in many cases of idiopathic a-fib. The beneficial effect of yoga and other alternative therapies is now being scientifically studied with encouraging results.

Acupressure /Acupuncture

Italian researchers looked at whether pressure points traditionally used in Traditional Chinese Medicine to treat palpitations would have any arrhythmic effects on paroxysmal and persistent a-fib. The treatment protocol consisted of 10, weekly acupuncture sessions focusing on the Neiguan,

Shenmen and Xinshu pressure points. In the first group of patients, individuals with permanent AF who had undergone successful cardioversion, puncturing of the Neiguan spot led to significantly lower rates of recurrence (35%) than in patients treated with no anti-arrhythmic drugs (54%) or sham acupuncture (69%). The low rates in recurrence seen in acupuncture are not significantly different to those in a group of patients treated with Amiodarone (27%). In selected patients with paroxysmal a-fib, acupuncture significantly reduced the duration and number of episodes. Whilst this was a relatively small study, the results are promising.

EFT or Emotional Freedom Technique is a form of acupressure which involves tapping with the fingertips over the energy meridians used in traditional acupuncture, whilst repeating positive affirmations. It is very simple to learn and I have heard of at least one patient who has been able to terminate an episode of a-fib using this technique. Typing Emotional Freedom Technique into any search engine will bring up a wealth of information.

How to Conquer your A-fib

1. Educate yourself about a-fib. Knowledge is power!
2. Seek proper advice from a qualified medical practitioner. Work with your personal physicians to tailor an individual treatment plan with regular reviews. Follow your physician's advice to ensure you are adequately anti-coagulated.
3. Ensure you are a healthy weight. The risk of developing a-fib increases with body mass!
4. Keep an a-fib diary. Note down everything you eat, drink, your activity level, stress level and anything else you think relevant. Then when you do get episodes you may be able to identify potential triggers.
5. Consider having a sleep study done to rule out obstructive sleep apnoea particularly if you are overweight or you snore
6. Check your thyroid levels
7. Get an oral hygiene check up to ensure there is no underlying infection.
8. Consider whether a vitamin or mineral deficiency could be contributing to your problem.
9. Rule out food triggers such as MSG, artificial sweeteners, gluten etc.
10. Consider being tested for H Pylori
11. Find support from other people on the same journey
12. Consider if alternative therapies such as yoga or acupuncture would be useful
13. Stress plays a big role in the disorder. Reduce stress as much as possible and consider an active stress management program.
14. Stay positive. Keeping a positive mental attitude reduces the burden of many chronic disorders –

including a-fib.

Above all realise that a-fib is treatable and beatable.

Stories of people who cured themselves of a-fib

To end this book, I would like to bring you three stories of people who have cured their a-fib by taking very different paths.

Patrick – Cured by Diet.

Patrick suffered from a-fib for approximately four years. The violent palpitations and lack of energy he suffered greatly affected the quality of his everyday life. Pat's episodes usually began at night just before he was about to fall asleep. "Suddenly I would be jolted awake" he explained. "My heart would take off at a mile a minute, skipping all over the place, jumping wild and crazy. The first time it happened I thought I was about to die".

Patrick was diagnosed with paroxysmal a-fib and mild hypertension. His episodes continued once or twice a week, and started to affect his quality of life. "I had trouble falling asleep at night as I worried about going into AF". Keeping a diary of his episodes, Patrick started to notice that they got worse after he ate certain foods. "At first I noticed it was when I ate at a certain restaurant a few blocks from my house. I would eat there a couple of times a week. It was mainly Asian food". It was only when I mentioned my symptoms to a friend who also ate there a lot that I started to make the connection". The friend suggested that Patrick may be sensitive to the MSG that the restaurant used in their cooking. "I didn't even know what Monosodium Glutamate was back then" Patrick admits. Back home, he started to research MSG. "What I read fitted in with my symptoms perfectly". Patrick quit eating at that particular restaurant and whilst his symptoms improved slightly, they didn't stop altogether.

"I consciously avoided eating all foods with MSG in them" he said, but he was still not out of the woods. "I became convinced that my a-fib was some sort of food reaction. I started to look into glutamate and other excitotoxins". What Patrick learned was he had an extreme reaction to all glutamate and that was responsible for his symptoms. "Overhauling my diet was tough. I avoided all processed food and switched to a caveman style of eating. I also supplemented with magnesium, taurine and co enzyme q10. The results were dramatic. Within a fortnight his a-fib had gone completely and its never come back.
"It was tough but worth the effort" Patrick says. "Being free of a-fib is awesome".

John – Cured By Catheter Ablation

John was a young athlete in his 20's when he had his first experience of a-fib. His transient attacks mainly started after intense workouts, however they were not caught on an event monitor, so they were merely labelled palpitations and he was told there was nothing to worry about. A few years passed and his a-fib appeared to come and go, his episodes were relatively short, just a few minutes at a time and didn't really have much of an impact on his life. He began endurance training and noticed his episodes would come as he was relaxing after training hard. He speculated it may have something to do with dehydration or electrolyte imbalance.

As time passed episodes got longer and nearer together. The frequent episodes were beginning to impact his life so he sought the advice of a cardiologist. He was referred to an EP, and after some discussion he decided that the best course of action would be catheter ablation. The procedure was scheduled for 3 months' time, and for John the ablation couldn't come soon enough.

Johns procedure took slightly longer than planned as the team found some atrial flutter that needed to be ablated. John awoke several hours later in perfect sinus rhythm.

It is normal after a catheter ablation for there to be some burst of a-fib and ectopic beats as the scar tissue is forming and the atria recover from the procedure. John experienced just a single burst of a-fib the day after the procedure which converted on its own in a couple of hours. That turned out to be his last ever episode of a-fib. Two years on he is still in normal sinus rhythm and the procedure was deemed a complete success.

Sam – Cured by Supplements

Sam suffered from panic and anxiety all of her life and she feels that led to the chronic magnesium deficiency which fuelled her a-fib. "Ever since I was young I suffered from debilitating panic – I would literally become frozen with fear. I started to suffer episodes of racing heart and palpitations in my teens. My doctor dismissed it as anxiety". As Sam entered her twenties her episodes got worse. "At that point I had no idea what it was that was causing these palpitations. I was so frightened that I thought I was on the verge of having a heart attack". Sam's diagnosis came when she had an episode of a-fib in her doctor's office. "They finally caught it on ECG. The sense of relief that it wasn't all in my head was immense". Sam was diagnosed with atrial fibrillation but doctors could find no explanation for it. "I decided to research the condition for myself. I found some research papers by Dr Carolyn Dean and information on magnesium deficiency which fitted my symptoms exactly".

"I bought some magnesium glycinate and the effects were noticeable almost straight away. I instantly felt calmer and could sleep better. I knew I was on to something immediately. I hadn't felt this good in years". Over the next few months as Sam's magnesium stores replenished her palpitations and skipped beats also subsided. "I couldn't believe how much better I felt, I must have been perilously low in magnesium for a long, long time". Sam also added taurine, vitamin c and vitamin b6 to her daily routine as a preventative measure. She remains a-fib free.

Made in United States
Troutdale, OR
06/22/2024

20749293R10046